C000161733

John Gunstone was a member of the Church of England's commission on the healing ministry and co-editor of its report, *A Time to Heal*. He is the author of *Healed, Restored, Forgiven–Liturgies, prayers and readings for the ministry of healing*, also published by the Canterbury Press.

After many years in parish and diocesan ministry, he is now Canon Emeritus of Manchester Cathedral.

Also by the same author

Healed, Restored, Forgiven

Liturgies and readings for the ministry of healing

A rich resource, full of gentle wisdom and realistic understanding, it provides prayers, readings and complete service outlines for use in a wide variety of pastoral situations. These include:

- personal prayers for the varying stages of an experience of illness or trouble
- prayers for intercessors
- prayers of preparation for healing services
- prayers for ministry teams
- a service of anointing with the laying on of hands
- a healing service within the Eucharist
- prayers of thanksgiving
- liturgies for the ministry of reconciliation
- an anthology of prayers, scripture passages and modern readings on the themes of healing, restoration and forgiveness.

Simplicity and versatility are maintained throughout, ensuring that the texts may be easily adapted for use in any setting – formal or informal, large or small.

1-85311-587-8   www.scm-canterburypress.co.uk

A TOUCHING PLACE

The healing ministry in the local church:
a practical handbook

John Gunstone

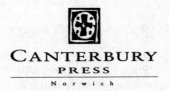

CANTERBURY
PRESS
Norwich

© John Gunstone 2005

First published in 2005 by the Canterbury Press Norwich
(a publishing imprint of Hymns Ancient & Modern Limited,
a registered charity)
St Mary's Works, St Mary's Plain, Norwich,
Norfolk, NR3 3BH

www.scm-canterburypress.co.uk

British Library Cataloguing in Publication data

A catalogue record for this book is available
from the British Library

ISBN 1-85311-631-9/9781-85311-631-5

Typeset by Regent Typesetting, London
Printed in Great Britain by
Bookmarque, Croydon, Surrey

Contents

To the lost Christ shows his face;
To the unloved he gives his embrace;
To those who cry in pain or disgrace,
Christ makes, with his friends, a touching place.

John L. Bell and Graham Maule

Introduction

This book is a guide for clergy and groups involved in healing services in church. I decided to write it from an Anglican viewpoint to avoid cluttering the text with alternative ecclesiastical titles (priest, minister, pastor, etc.). I hope readers from other traditions will tolerate this; they should not, I think, have much difficulty in relating what I have said to their own church structures.

Groups who offer prayers for healing are variously known as 'prayer ministry teams', 'healing groups', 'intercessors for the sick', and so on. I have chosen to call them 'healing prayer teams'. Since the healing ministry is rooted in prayer, this title indicates what their purpose is – to pray with others for healing. It also avoids giving the impression that those who belong to it are to be regarded as 'healers'. Individual members of such teams, whether they are clergy or laity, I have entitled 'ministers'.

Then there is the matter of what to call those to whom they minister. 'The ones receiving ministry' is rather a mouthful. I discarded 'clients' as unsatisfactory, and I certainly did not relish being politically correct and referring to them as 'customers' or even 'consumers'! In the end I settled for 'suppliants', for this is what they are – individuals seeking God's grace through the prayers of their sisters and brothers in Christ.

Writers are confronted with the problem of how to refer to the two sexes jointly in pronouns. To keep referring in print to 'him or her' and 'his or hers' is tiresome. (It was easier when Anglican clergy were all male!) I have therefore adopted the device of using the plural pronoun, 'they' and 'theirs', even when the subject of the sentence is singular. Only where this might be confusing have I resorted to using the singular pronouns separately.

I have not attempted to discuss the theological and pastoral problems which can surround the ministry of healing. Here I am only concerned with the practicalities of gathering, training and supervising a team as it begins to exercise its ministry during services in church. These wider issues are discussed very comprehensively in the Church of England's report, *A Time to Heal* (Church House Publishing, 2000).

This book is intended as a companion to my *Healed, Restored, Forgiven* (Canterbury Press, 2004), which contains prayers, services and readings for both ministry teams and suppliants involved in the healing ministry.

John Gunstone

I

HEALING IN CHURCH LIFE TODAY

Chapter Summary

- Healing in the Church's history.
- Developments in the last hundred years.
- Revival of sacramental and charismatic ministries to the sick.
- Movements which have influenced these developments.
- Initiatives by individuals and groups in different denominations.
- Involvement of increasing numbers of lay persons as well as clergy.

From the days when Peter and John healed the lame man at the Beautiful Gate of the temple (Acts 3.1–10), and the elders prayed, anointed and laid hands on the sick (James 5.14–16), the Church has always had a ministry of healing. Throughout the centuries Christians have believed that the healing work of Jesus Christ continues by his Spirit through his people who pray for the sick in his name.

To appreciate the ways in which the Church exercises that ministry today, we have to look back briefly at the traditional practice of it among congregations. The sick were – and, of course, still are – remembered by name during the intercessions in church services, and visited and prayed with at home and in hospital. Those who are regular communicants have the sacrament taken to them. This ministry is normally a priest- or pastor-centred affair, though of course members of the laity are involved in caring for the sick at home and in hospital. The general assumption of nearly everybody in the older denominations has been that the actual healing of individuals was the business of the caring professions; the Church's job was to support these professionals and their patients with appropriate intercessions.

However, during the last hundred years developments have taken place that have resulted in the Church becoming more directly involved in the healing processes, principally through anointing and the laying on of hands with prayer invoking the healing grace of God. This has become increasingly common among all the denominations, not only in Britain but in other parts of the world. It is exercised privately in small groups as well as in public services.

Encouragement for these developments came from various sources. News of how the healing ministry was exercised among the Holiness and Pentecostal people in America spread over the Atlantic to influence supporters of the Keswick Convention and others in the Free Churches. Anglo-Catholic teaching on the centrality of the sacraments (including anointing of the sick) affected the thought and practice of the Anglican Church. Among Roman Catholics the liturgical movement, with its interest in the continuity of the Church of the Bible with the Church of today, caused increasing numbers to question why the use of anointing was restricted to the last rites for the dying when in the New Testament it is clearly associated with healing.

The result was that individuals began to take initiatives to restore practices such as prayer with the laying on of hands.

I only have space to mention a few of the names of these; they are representative of dozens of others, well known or little known, who influenced the healing ministry in their own denominations and beyond. They pioneered the wider ministry of healing with which we are becoming familiar.

The Revd Percy Dearmer, vicar of St Mary's, Primrose Hill, Hampstead, formed the ecumenical Guild of Health and published services for anointing and the laying on of hands in *The Parson's Handbook* (1907) – services that were promoted in the Church of England by the Guild of St Raphael, founded in 1915. James Moore Hickson, an Anglican layman, set up the Divine Healing Mission in 1905 and was commended for his work by Randall Davidson, the Archbishop of Canterbury. Another Anglican, Dorothy Kerin, convinced she had been miraculously healed after a near-terminal illness in 1911, began praying for the sick with the laying on of hands and built up a network of supporters that ultimately led to the foundation of the Christian Centre for Health Care and Ministry at Burrswood in Sussex after the Second World War.

During the inter-war years the preaching and writing of the Methodist Leslie Weatherhead did much to help the Church to realize the link between psychology, the individual and psychotherapy in healing; perhaps more than any other clergyman of his generation he inspired later advances in Christian counselling. J. Cameron Peddie, a Presbyterian minister in Glasgow, exercised a remarkable ministry of healing and told his story in *The Forgotten Talent* (1942) – one of the first of many such books that were to be published in the following years.

Advised by its liturgical scholars, the Second Vatican Council (1962–65) decreed that anointing was to be used not only as a preparation for death but also as a sacrament for the healing of those who are seriously ill, and arranged for appropriate services to be drawn up for this purpose. Prominent among those who followed this up was the American, Fr Francis MacNutt, who in his teaching advocated the practice of 'soaking prayer' with the sick; his book *Healing*, first published in the 1970s, sold over a million copies worldwide.

In 1958 a commission set up by the Archbishops of Canterbury and York produced a report, *The Church's Ministry of Healing*, drawn up by a large panel of clergy and representatives of the British Medical Association. Among other things, it made practical suggestions on organizing public services at which hands were laid on individuals for healing. In making those suggestions the report was prophetic, for when it was published few clergy and even fewer lay people imagined they would be involved in such a ministry during their Sunday services in 20 or 30 years' time.

In the 1960s and 1970s the healing ministry was greatly influenced by the charismatic renewal. This movement owed much to the teaching of individual Pentecostal pastors like David Du Plessis, who were willing to share their experiences of the Holy Spirit and his gifts with those in other denominations. Central to their message, expounded from relevant scripture passages and illustrated by personal testimonies, was the belief that Christians should not only be saved in the name of Jesus but should also be baptized in the Holy Spirit. Then they – laity as well as clergy – would receive 'the Father's promise' and be 'clothed with power from on high' (Luke 24.49) to exercise gifts of the Holy Spirit (charisms) for the building up of the Church (1 Corinthians 12.14).

At first it was the experience of being baptized in the Spirit that attracted most attention, especially if accompanied by speaking in tongues. Although Pentecostal doctrines about Spirit-baptism were much debated, nevertheless the charismatic renewal awakened among many a desire to pray and to exercise the Spirit's gifts. The lists of these charisms in the New Testament offered a portrait of a Church in which every member was equipped by the Holy Spirit to serve as Christ's disciples. These gifts of healing were obviously relevant to so many people's needs.

Leaders in the renewal taught how the healing ministry could be developed through gifts of discernment, words of knowledge and wisdom, deliverance from evil and evidence of physical healing. One of these leaders was John Wimber, a former rock musician, who founded the Vineyard churches in California and who was introduced to this country by David Watson. During visits to cities and conference centres in the early 1980s, he taught that Jesus' ministry of healing was a manifestation of the Kingdom of God. He said that the contemporary Church, like the apostles in the book of Acts, should continue to preach that gospel in expectation that 'signs and wonders' of the Holy Spirit's presence and power would be manifested among those who heard it.

Certain aspects of Wimber's ministry were controversial, though what he said was sometimes misreported. Wimber himself was humble about his healing gifts (his son died of cancer when he was at the height of his ministry, and Wimber died of the same disease himself a few years later). What was memorable about his teaching method was that he not only spoke about the healing ministry but demonstrated openly how it was done and involved his audiences in it.

Consequently his sessions were novel experiences in religious education. After leading worship and giving his talk, Wimber invited individuals to come forward and receive prayer with the laying on of hands. While the members of his team ministered to them, he stood on one side and gave a running commentary on what was happening. When the demonstration was over, Wimber divided his audience into twos and threes and told them to pray for one another. That was a shock for those who had never done such a thing before! But many were surprised to discover how easy it was to do this once they had recovered from their initial embarrassment. They were also mildly surprised to find that at these meetings they were frequently sharing in prayer with Christians of a different denomination from their own who happened to be sitting near them.

True, some of those who testified they were healed at these sessions did not seem to show signs of it; but there were others who said the ministry they had received had been a significant factor in their cure. But that did not prevent these demonstrations from making a powerful impact on the audience, laity and clergy alike. Many of them returned home with a vision of how they could initiate such a ministry in their own congregations.

Other agencies influenced by the charismatic renewal also helped to project and broaden this vision. The Fountain Trust, founded to promote the lessons of the renewal among the mainstream denominations, included ministry to the sick in its meetings and conferences. The healing ministry became a popular topic at national ecumenical gatherings like Spring Harvest and New Wine. Bodies such as the Acorn Christian Healing Trust were founded. Numerous books were published on the subject, often containing personal testimonies. News and articles appeared in Christian newspapers and periodicals; for several years there was a magazine called *Healing and Wholeness*.

So the vision of the Church that preaches the gospel in the expectation that spiritual gifts of healing will be manifested began to spread, and with it there emerged teams of laity trained to share in that ministry with their clergy.

It was because of these developments that the bishops of the Church of England commissioned a new report in 2000. *A Time to Heal* was compiled by a group representing the caring professions and clergy and laity with experience in ministry to the sick. It consulted widely to draw together information on how the ministry is practised both at home and abroad among the various denominations today. It discusses a wide range of related matters, such as co-operation with health authorities, complementary and alternative therapies, and deliverance from evil. Among other things, it recommends that dioceses should appoint advisers whose task it is to help parishes develop their ministry.

But what is notable about this report, in contrast to the 1958 one, is that the role of the laity is fully recognized, especially the role they play in prayer healing teams, and it makes recommendations about these developments. In this book I've suggested how these might be followed up in the life and mission of a local church of any denomination – with allowances, as I said in the Introduction, for the limitations of my Anglican approach to the subject.

For Discussion

- What experience have you had personally of the Church's healing ministry?
- Have you been to a service in which the ministry of healing was offered?

2

How to Begin

Chapter Summary

- Key role of the clergy in developing the healing ministry in congregations.
- Opportunities to learn through the experiences as well as through meetings and literature.
- Preparing a congregation for developments through systematic teaching.

One day a vicar rang me up and asked me if I would come to a meeting in his parish. He was having problems, he said, with a group of young church members. They were urging him to start healing services and he did not know how to deal with them. He'd been told that I had some experience in the healing ministry, and he thought it would help if I could meet them.

I duly turned up one evening at his vicarage and was taken by his wife into a sitting room where half a dozen men and women, mostly in their twenties, were sitting. After she had introduced me, the wife said her husband had been delayed but would join us shortly. She then left the room.

During the next few minutes I discovered that the group had been on a Christian holiday conference where they had learned about the ministry of healing. They had come back wanting to start such a ministry in their church, and believed there were many in the congregation who would welcome it. I gathered the vicar wasn't keen but had agreed with their request to seek advice.

At that point the vicar came into the room, apologizing for the delay. I gave a talk on the scriptural basis for the ministry and its development in recent years. This was followed by questions and a discussion. I do not remember all that was said, but it was obvious to me that the vicar, though he said very little, found the enthusiasm of the young people difficult to handle.

After an hour or so, it was time for me to go. The vicar escorted me outside to my car and, as he shook my hand, said wearily, 'Thanks for coming. I don't think we shall be having healing services in my church. You see, I have theological problems about this healing business.'

I admired his concern for the young people and his willingness to invite me to meet them, but I drove home feeling sad that an opportunity to harness their enthusiasm for the cause of the Kingdom was being lost. With proper teaching and supervision they might have added much to the mission of the Church in his parish. I was not surprised to hear some months later that the group had left his church and gone to worship elsewhere. I never met him or them again.

I tell this story because it illustrates a lesson of experience that, in nine cases out of ten, it is almost impossible for the ministry of a healing prayer team to be introduced into a congregation without the support of the priest or those in pastoral leadership. This is true of any church, whatever its denomination or tradition.

I should, however, point out that priests have another reason to be careful about introducing this ministry to their parishes. Lay involvement is a welcome development; it releases gifts and graces in different people that would otherwise be dormant. But without proper training and supervision things can go badly wrong. When an over-enthusiastic group is insensitive in praying with and laying hands on people, they can cause hurt and disappointment. Then it is usually the priest who gets the blame for allowing them such freedom.

On the other hand, things can also go wrong if it is the priest himself who is over-enthusiastic and tries to introduce new forms of the ministry without preparing the congregation for them. A typical scenario is when priests go to a conference, hear stories of miraculous healings and experience blessings themselves. They come back to their parishes zealous to introduce prayer with the laying on of hands for healing into the services the following Sunday.

A full frontal presentation of charismatic teachings and practices of this ministry is difficult for traditional church folk to take. A few may appreciate what their priests are trying to do, but the rest react with suspicion and hostility. As a result the congregation are divided. It may take one or two years before they are ready to consider the healing ministry again. This is a pity, for Anglicans and those in the traditional churches are far more open to the healing ministry nowadays than they were a generation ago. They hear about it through programmes on radio and television, they attend healing services in other churches, and they talk to others who have had experience of this ministry.

To describe one strategy for introducing the ministry of healing, I will imagine I am the vicar of a parish where the pastoral care of the sick has been exercised in the traditional Anglican way from time immemorial. Sick people have appreciated it when I've visited them and taken them Communion. Some have told me they thought they got better more quickly as a result. At a recent diocesan synod I attended with two representatives from my church, a speaker introduced the report *A Time to Heal* and the bishop presided over a healing service at which many went forward for ministry. At the synod I met a couple of clergy from neighbouring parishes who told me they have begun arranging such services in their churches and plan to form healing prayer teams to assist them.

On the way home from the synod I discussed with my companions what we had learned. Their reactions were different. One, a woman, was quite interested in what she heard and saw; the other, a man, said he didn't think the parish was ready for such services yet. They both agreed, however, that I should gradually introduce teaching about the healing ministry to the congregation and await reactions.

I realized, however, that I needed to be better informed myself on the theological basis of the healing ministry and how it can be expressed in the pastoral strategy of an English parish church. After making enquiries, I learned that there was to be a short residential conference on the subject and I booked myself a place on it. While I was there, I listened to lectures, joined in discussion groups, and received prayer for a minor ailment that had been troubling me for months. I took part in a healing service which ended the conference and returned home, armed with a couple of books I had been recommended and feeling better equipped to teach the congregation about this ministry.

I try to pray for guidance that I may be able to introduce the idea of a healing ministry to the congregation in a sensitive manner to gain their interest and support. I also test my ideas by reading Chapter 14 of *A Time to Heal*, which discusses the pastoral basis of developing the healing ministry in a parish.

I begin by discussing it in casual one-to-one conversations with various members as opportunities arise. I make a special point of talking to those whose support I will need when I promote the idea publicly – the churchwardens, lay leaders and persons who are respected for their wisdom. I guess that in this way news of my interest in the healing ministry will become a subject of gossip on the parochial grapevine and give me a chance to assess reactions.

Without making the ministry the topic of every sermon and church meeting, I introduce it using whatever means of communication I have to teach about it. My monthly vicar's letter in the parish magazine is a useful vehicle for this; so is the church bookstall, which I stock with books, magazines, tapes and CDs for enquirers.

Gradually certain members of the congregation start asking me questions, especially those who feel they need the healing ministry themselves. When several have raised the issue, I report this to the churchwardens and parochial church council and suggest that we (involving them as well as myself!) organize a conference on a weekday evening or a Saturday and invite the vicar of a neighbouring parish where a healing ministry has been established to come and speak, bringing a few members of his healing prayer team with him to share their experiences.

Preparing the congregation in this way gives opportunities for those who have doubts and questions to express them and seek reassurance and answers. People are deterred for all sorts of personal reasons – genuine misunderstandings, bad experiences of this ministry in the past, a mindset over-influenced by our scientific culture, and fears of what might happen. There will probably be always a few who will not accept ideas that are new to them; I need to take care in the weeks and months to come to see that they do not feel excluded if the healing ministry develops in the parish.

After the conference and various other meetings, the parochial church council agrees that I should explore the possibility of developing the healing ministry along the lines described at the conference.

What the next step should be depends on local circumstances. In the following chapter I will continue in my role as an imaginary vicar who wishes to gather together a healing prayer team. But in many parishes it may be best to begin by arranging a simple service of prayers for healing one weekday evening.

This is what I did when I was a parish priest (I am now speaking about my personal experiences). I invited those who wanted prayer for healing to come to church with a friend on Wednesday evenings once a month. The service consisted of a scripture reading, a brief homily, intercessory prayers for the sick and those who looked after them, and a short form of confession.

Then I invited suppliants to come and kneel at the communion rail with their friends beside them. I laid hands on them and prayed according to their needs. I asked the friend to pray for them, too; most did this silently, but in time one or two followed me in praying aloud.

The numbers who came were never large. I think 12 was the maximum. But it remained a regular item in the parish programme until I left a couple of years later, and I'm glad to say that my successor continued the service.

During these years various people were helped, and a few declared that the ministry had been a vital factor in healing their ailments. Looking back, I can see that my invitation to bring a friend to these services was a first step in introducing the practice of ministering in pairs. The friend who knelt with a suppliant became a partner in prayer with me for a few moments. I didn't realize it at the time – and I'm sure the friend didn't – but I was unconsciously moving towards the New Testament pattern of ministering in pairs.

For Discussion

- When did you last hear or speak about the healing ministry in a sermon or in a discussion?
- Which one of Jesus Christ's healing miracles interests you most?

3

GATHERING THE TEAM

Chapter Summary

- A team of trained lay persons an important resource for a congregation's healing ministry.
- Discerning and encouraging those who believe they may be called by God.
- Testing their motivations and gifts.
- Commitment to prayer and working in a team.

The decision to form a healing prayer team has to be made with the same care as choosing licensed readers, pastoral assistants or group elders. If the team is to function properly, it will be sharing in that pastoral care of people for which the parish priest is ultimately responsible. It needs, therefore, to be undergirded with the same prayer that led to the developments outlined in the last chapter.

Continuing my imaginary role as the vicar of a parish, I begin to wonder how I should start recruiting a team. Should I make an announcement in church one Sunday, inviting anyone who is interested in being a member to let me know? Or should I wait and see who shows an interest before taking any initiative personally?

On reflection I decide that the second option is better. I've been teaching the congregation about the ministry for some weeks now, and I've been praying about its development in the parish. So I should expect God to be stirring the hearts of those whom he is calling to serve in such a team. And this is what he does. The response comes as individuals approach me with comments and questions.

I've heard from my friends in London that they help at healing services in their church.

I've often felt I'd like to pray with sick neighbours when I've called on them, but I'm not sure what I should say.

Ever since I read that book on healing you lent me, I've wondered if the Lord might want me to be more involved in it.

We used to have healing services nearly every Sunday at the Pentecostal church we went to when we lived in Chile. Surely the Holy Spirit could heal here as he did out there?

I don't regard everyone who approaches me in this way as a potential team member. Most people are concerned about health – their own as well as others' – and they usually welcome opportunities to talk about it with the vicar. But further conversation with them helps me to see if their concern about health includes learning how to pray for others as well as themselves. Eventually I sense that three or four of those I have talked to come into this category, and I suggest we meet to discuss the matter further.

I've been warned that I should be cautious of individuals who tell me confidently that God has given them a gift of healing and that he is calling them to exercise that gift in church. There are, I understand, a few 'spiritual gypsies' who roam round different churches claiming they are 'healers' and depart when they have caused trouble through their insensitivity. So if the one coming to me with such claims has only recently joined the congregation, I get in touch with the pastoral leadership of their former church to seek advice about them.

If the report I receive is favourable, then I welcome them in the hope that we can benefit from their previous experiences. But if it is unfavourable, I tactfully tell them that I would prefer the congregation got to know them better before they joined the team. I then wait to see if they stay with us or take themselves with their gifts elsewhere!

At the opposite extreme are modest individuals who are too shy to think of offering themselves. However, their friends may know they are already quietly exercising a simple ministry to the sick and suggest their names to me. I take such suggestions seriously; they may be instances of how the Holy Spirit prompts a group of Christians to discern spiritual gifts in one another.

This, then, is the way my imaginary vicar began forming a team. There are, however, other matters that require consideration.

Members of the caring professions in congregations are usually interested when the Church's ministry of healing is being discussed. Christian nurses and other carers are often willing to join a team, though many doctors are hesitant. The latter are often unsure – and understandably so – how prayer and the laying on of hands relates to their role in a secular and scientific health service; they are also cautious about being involved in anything that might be regarded as an extension of their professional responsibilities.

But not all are like that. I once had a conversation with a doctor in general practice about the healing ministry. He was a Methodist local preacher and confessed that he had often wished he could pray and lay hands on people when he saw their needs. I suggested that the next time he preached he should do just that.

I did not see him for some weeks, but when we next met the first thing he said to me was that he had followed my advice on the previous Sunday. He had been preaching in a church in another circuit. At the end of his sermon he had cautiously offered to pray and lay hands on any who needed healing. To his astonishment, many came forward. When I asked how he felt about it afterwards, I remember his words for he said them with such feeling: 'John, for the first time in my life I felt totally fulfilled as a doctor!'

In the process of gathering our team, one or two may tell us that they are interested in the ministry of healing, but after a discussion they reveal that they are really more concerned about seeking healing (of all kinds) for themselves rather than ministering to others. Though we should not necessarily dissuade such individuals, they may not be very reliable as members of a team. But unless they show signs of emotional problems or mental disorders requiring professional help, by joining the team they can provide an opportunity for other members to learn how to minister to such needs. In my experience, troubled individuals like these either cease to attend team meetings, or they are so thankful to be helped that they are able to minister to others. Indeed, it is those who have known the healing power of God in their own lives who are usually the most faithful in praying for healing for others.

None of us comes to any meeting – and certainly not meetings about the healing ministry – without some personal agenda. Even those who join a team because they believe God is calling them, bring with them needs that one day they may share with the rest of the team. Adapting the dictum that a Christian is a beggar who can tell other beggars where to find bread, we might describe ourselves on the team as those who know their own need of healing and who want to help others to find it.

Ideally, members of a team should be those Christians who are growing in their faith in the Lord Jesus as their Saviour and Healer. Since the team's main purpose is prayer, it is not the place for those who are unwilling to accept a discipline of becoming pray-ers. They should also be comfortable working in a team under the pastoral authority of the priest, and self-aware enough to realize their own personal limitations.

They should be willing to meet regularly with others, to pray with them, to share our own needs and experiences, and to accept that we never cease to be students in this ministry. And they must be willing to be corrected when necessary. There will be times when we have to repent for mistakes and failures before God and apologize to others. But such errors help to keep us humble. They remind us of our human weaknesses and of our role of unworthy servants of the Great Physician.

Yet the healing ministry can be rewarding. Like other ministries in the Body of Christ, members with different gifts find that when they work together their united ministry is more powerful in the Holy Spirit than the sum total of those gifts added together. And when a suppliant comes up one day and says how much the Lord has healed them through your ministry, you experience of little leap of heavenly joy.

In many churches there already exist groups who meet regularly to pray for the sick and are involved in things like hospital visiting and shopping for the housebound. But if not all the members want to engage personally in this development of the healing ministry, they can continue their meetings with a special intention of praying for the team in its work.

I realize that there are congregations in which the formation of a healing prayer team may be a good deal more haphazard than I have outlined here. Priests in small churches may not be able at first to think of a single person who could be recruited. They may have to be content with the kind of simple service I described in Chapter 2. But I think it is likely that, if they persist in prayer and in exercising this ministry as opportunities arise, they will eventually discover that the Spirit moves people – including one or two of the most unlikely ones – to become involved with them in it. God can, and often does, surprise us.

For Discussion

- Have you ever been in a situation in which you wished you could pray for healing with another person, but couldn't?
- If you had been able to pray for healing with another person, what would have been your real motive?

4

TRAINING THE TEAM

Chapter Summary

- Regularity of team meetings.
- Programme for initial and ongoing training for: spiritual formation, personal relationships, listening, scripture and doctrine, practical exercises.

One way of looking at a healing prayer team is to see it as a Christian expression of the kind of teams within which those in the caring professions are used to working – teams in hospital wards, operating theatres and emergency departments, in health care centres and in nursing homes. And, like these, our teams have similar needs.

The team in the caring professions needs leadership which is itself accountable to a superior authority. Within the team are those with different but complementary skills and experiences. Team meetings for training, planning and mutual support are needed if its members are to serve the patients effectively. Members have to learn to work together and respect each other's roles. Specialists and consultants have to be called in to deal with particular cases. And then there are teams of social workers and others who are responsible for the follow-up of the patients, to see that they are able to resume a normal life once their therapy is completed.

The fact that those in the caring professions are in paid employment and those in healing prayer teams are usually volunteers does not alter these needs. Both require the same framework within which to serve the individuals who come to them. The real difference is that the members of the healing prayer team are united in the faith that they are called to serve others by the Lord who will empower them by his Spirit for his work among people. (That may be true of individual Christians in teams of caring professionals, of course, but it is not usually true of everyone in them.)

The priest will usually be the trainer of the team to begin with because, as I have said, he is ultimately responsible for the pastoral care of the congregation (and, in the Anglican Church, answerable to his bishop). In time there may be others with whom this task can be shared or to whom it can be delegated; when this happens the priest has to be satisfied that what is being taught and practised is orthodox and acceptable.

Various Christian bodies publish training courses for the healing ministry. The diocesan adviser should have an up-to-date list of them. Roger Vaughan's *Saints Alive! Healing in the Church* a good starter. *In Search of Wholeness* by Russ Parker, Derek Fraser and David Rivers is comprehensive and student-friendly. *A Time to Heal* gives a wide overview of the ministry, with advice on paths and pitfalls; it was not designed to be a training manual but it is very useful for general reference purposes.

Team training covers various topics.

Spiritual formation. Our basic relationship in Christian ministry, as in Christian living, is with the Lord God. Unless the members are willing to learn more about this relationship and to practise it in their personal prayer life, they will be less able to minister faithfully in his name. They may be helpful at a human level, but such help as they give will remain at that human level unless God in his sovereignty transforms it with his grace.

Members will be at different stages in their spiritual development, and their experiences will be very varied. We should not try and force them into a particular pattern but enable them to develop the relationship they already have with God. Because this is so important, I have discussed it in the next two chapters.

Personal relationships. Understanding how we relate to others through the experience of team membership provides another learning opportunity. As members grow to trust one another and to share personal matters at team meetings, they become more aware of what lies behind their own motivations and reactions. This does not mean that team meetings become informal group therapy sessions, but something of the value of such sessions can be part of the learning process.

Listening. We need to learn to listen to God, but we also have to learn to listen to those who come to us for prayer. During the healing ministry in a church service there may only be a minute or so for them to tell us what the trouble is; but what they say and the way they say it are pointers in discerning how we should pray for them. Courses on Christian Listening such as those run by the Acorn Trust are useful add-ons to training the team.

Scripture and doctrine. Members should be encouraged to become more familiar with the scriptures, especially those passages that are building blocks for Christian theologies of suffering and healing. There is great value in reading some scripture at all team meetings, even if only for a few minutes' reflection on a verse or two.

The Bible reveals that healing is a sign of the salvation that comes from God the Father through the Son in the power of the Holy Spirit, and that we were initiated into that healing and saving grace at our baptism. The introduction to the liturgies of Christian initiation in *Common Worship* has a brief but admirable summary of this truth; it can form the basis of discussions on what baptism means for each one of us and how it is the foundation of the healing ministry.

The New Testament uses the term healing both for physical healing and for the broader salvation that Jesus brings. But in this ministry we have to recognize that we may receive God's grace in different ways: sometimes as an experience of being healed, but at other times through the strength he gives in bearing our weaknesses. Wise teachers remind their students that this ministry, like all ministries, begins at the foot of the Cross.

History and tradition. The story of the Church's healing ministry through the centuries is instructive; there is much in it that helps us to see the relevance of contemporary teaching and practice as well as to avoid the errors of the past. Among the lessons from the past are the right use of the sacraments and the spiritual gifts in this ministry, and the role of the ministry within the mission of the Church.

Caring professions. In training we should allow time to look at the changing values and attitudes to health and healing in our contemporary society. People in the western world feel that they have a right to health until they die; they expect every illness and disability to be cured with the rapid advances in medicine and paramedical practices.

Certainly it is important that those of us who pray with and minister to others for healing recognize and respect all these other agencies for health and healing, and to see in them – as far as possible within the boundaries of Christian ethics (not always an easy task of discernment) – the workings of the same Spirit that we seek through prayers and sacramental signs. Yet the Church's ministry remains distinctive from them in that its ultimate aim is the glory of God.

Teams must respect the work of those in the caring professions whether they are Christians or not. No Anglican teacher I know has ever echoed those extremists who warn suppliants that to go to a doctor after receiving prayer for healing is a sign of a lack of faith. The contemporary Church is sometimes critical of certain advances in scientific medicine, but we do not doubt that the caring professions are responsible for marvellous cures and palliative treatments (even though they, like the rest of us, make mistakes at times). There should never be an occasion when we advise suppliants to give up their medication without first consulting their doctor.

Members should be aware of complementary and alternative therapies. There is a large and expanding market for these, and it is not always easy to discern which are acceptable for Christians and which they should be advised to avoid. There is a detailed description of these therapies in Chapter 10 of *A Time to Heal*.

Practical exercises. Training needs to include practical demonstrations on how to lay hands on a suppliant, either as an individual minister or as one of a pair, and on how to anoint. Instruction on how individuals receive the ministry of reconciliation and on how the bread and wine of the Eucharist are administered may also be useful.

When I first began praying for individuals for healing I used to lay my hands lightly on their heads – one hand across their forehead and the other at the back, rather as I would hold a football. But I have since become more flexible. Some suppliants find hands on their head uncomfortable; others have hairstyles that prohibit it! Now I often place a hand on a shoulder instead. With those lying in bed, especially in a hospital ward, I simply hold a hand. When I anoint, I make a small cross with my finger on the forehead.

During the course of training one or two members may spontaneously present personal problems and request prayer for them. With their permission the instructor can use these requests as a means of a demonstrating how to minister to one another. He or she invites another member to join in the prayer for the suppliant, with explanations afterwards. Later in the course the instructor might invite two of the team to minister to their friend under direction, rather as I described John Wimber did in his sessions (see Chapter 1). I must stress, however, that this must be done sensitively; much depends on how well the instructor knows the members concerned and at what stage in the course such opportunities arise.

This list of topics looks formidable, but it is not presented as a possible syllabus for the first few sessions! Rather, the list opens up areas that might be explored by the team during its meetings in the months and years after it has been established. As we shall see in Chapter 7, training remains a regular item on the agenda of team meetings. In this way members are constantly refreshed and do not become trapped in casual routine through over-familiarity.

At what point are the members proficient enough to embark on a public ministry in a service? That is a decision which must be left to the priest or instructor. The members themselves may begin to sense when they are ready for this next step. The way they have related to one another and ministered to one another during the course can be an indicator.

Yet in one sense we are never fully trained. And we shall make mistakes – and hopefully, learn from them, too. But if the congregation has been informed that the team is preparing to pray with individuals who request it we can be reasonably sure that they will understand if things do not go as smoothly as we had hoped.

In some congregations teams are commissioned at a special service (rather as choir persons, wardens, parochial church council members and others are). Much depends on the customs and outlook of each congregation. Personally, I prefer not to make the ministry of the team too formal a structure, merely printing their names in the church's publications from time to time, so that everyone knows who they are.

For Discussion

- Which of the training topics listed in this chapter do you think is the most important?
- Are there other occasions besides team meetings (during sermons, groups, courses, etc.) when you have heard any of the training topics explained or discussed?

5

THE PRAYER OF INTERCESSION

Chapter Summary

- Prayer as conscious awareness of and response to God's presence.
- Relating to the Three Persons of the Holy Trinity in intercession.
- An act of the will enriched by controlled emotion.
- Learning about prayer from traditional formularies.

Since intercessions are at the heart of the team's ministry, I want to examine those aspects of it that have a particular relevance to the healing ministry. In this chapter I will discuss the nature of intercessory prayer and in the next chapter the prayers of two people when they minister together as members of a team.

Prayer may be defined as our conscious response to the love that God the Father offers to us in Jesus Christ. It springs from our awareness of God's presence and the beginnings of our desire to communicate with him. That is why in traditional spirituality it has been called the practice of the presence of God.

Often, of course, we are not always aware of his presence. Christians can grow into a discipline of making acts of recollection whenever and wherever they are, but normally we are so immersed in our everyday activities and interests that our thoughts are elsewhere. It is when we do recollect God's presence and he becomes the focus of our reverent attention that prayer begins.

Many Christians commence their prayers by saying, 'In the Name of the Father, and of the Son, and of the Holy Spirit' – perhaps also making the sign of the cross. That salutation is a reminder that when we pray our relationship is with the Holy Trinity, the Three Persons in the One Godhead.

This classic doctrine of the mystery of God's Being was formed in the first Christian centuries, as the Church's bishops and teachers meditated on what the Bible reveals about God and his redeeming work and on their own experiences of faith, worship and discipleship. That led them at various councils to declare that God is one, but that in his Being there are three Persons – not three individuals, but three modes or forms in which his divine Being exists.

The words they used, which have become familiar through reciting the Creeds – 'Being' (or 'Substance') and 'Persons' – were borrowed from the language of contemporary Greek philosophy. In those years Hellenism was the dominant culture of the lands in which the gospel spread and it provided a vocabulary for Christian teachers and Church councils as they sought the Holy Spirit's guidance in defending the doctrine of God from various heresies.

Ultimately, of course, God's Being is far beyond our comprehension. But it is important to realize that when we pray we are in conversation with God who is a Tri-Unity of Three Persons; or, to adapt one of Paul's prayers, that we are yielding in faith to 'the grace of the Lord Jesus Christ, the love of God, and the fellowship of the Holy Spirit' (2 Corinthians 13.13). As one of the early Fathers put it, although God is one he is not solitary.

One way of approaching the mystery is to consider how many people have come to have faith in God through the order of the Persons of the Trinity named in the passage just quoted (though Paul was not conscious he was laying down one of the scriptural foundations for this doctrine; it was later that the Church realized it was the apostle's inspiration that led him to express his prayer in this way).

A person's faith often begins with an increasing interest in the Jesus of the Gospels. This happens in different ways – reading the Bible and Christian literature; conversations with believers or enquirers; visits to churches and places of pilgrimage; artistic representations of Christ in pictures, sculptures, drama and films; music; attendance at worship and missions; and times of crisis in their personal lives.

These experiences lead them to think about Jesus' relationship with his Father, especially the love of God manifested in his life, death and resurrection. Slowly they begin to realize that the Jesus of the Gospels was – and is – the Son of God, sharing in the divine nature of the Father. So Paul's phrases 'the grace of the Lord Jesus Christ' and 'the love of God' are unfolded with new meaning for them. Through Christ they begin to think about their relationship with God the Father. The Lord's Prayer, which they may have known (and probably said) since childhood, begins to come alive for them.

But then they are led to realize that this 'coming alive' is more than an intellectual assent to Christ's teaching or a deep feeling of wondering admiration. It is a stirring of God's Holy Spirit deep within them, moving them to respond to the grace that Christ offers them and the love which the Father has for them. The result is the birth of a conviction that they are within 'the fellowship of the Holy Spirit', which finds its chief expression in the Church of God. Confirmation of this comes when they begin to experience the fruit and the gifts of the Spirit in themselves and in other Christians.

Having said this, I should add that God moves among human beings in an infinite variety of different ways to bring people to himself. There is no set order or stereotyped pattern. But it often proves to be the case that Christ's grace is the doorway to men and women's realization of the Father's love and the Spirit's fellowship.

All this is received sacramentally when converts are baptized in the name of the Holy Trinity, renouncing evil, confessing their sins, declaring their faith in Jesus Christ as their Lord and Saviour, and receiving the Holy Spirit (or when they reaffirm these things if they were baptized as children). So our new life began when we became God's children by adoption and grace; and prayer is central to that new life if we are to continue in it.

Like all relationships, prayer is varied and enriching. It may begin with acts of confession, petition, thanksgiving and praise. It may lead to reflection on what God's word means for us today. It may develop into periods of silent contemplation and adoration. But prayer is essentially a movement of the Holy Spirit creating within us a desire to respond to God's love – and all that follows from that, including the ministry of healing.

Many times we may not feel anything when we pray. That is not an uncommon experience among Christians. Even the great teachers of the spiritual life went through times of spiritual dryness. But feelings are not reliable signs of the reality of our response. Prayer begins and ends with an act of will, not a wave of emotion. Indeed, we should be suspicious of anyone or anything which aims to manipulate our emotions as we try to pray.

That does not mean, however, that we should attempt to quash our feelings. If our response to God is to be real, it should be a response of the whole of ourselves – beginning with our wills but including our emotions as well as our body, mind and spirit. God's love demands of us nothing less. The Law of Moses recognized this, and Jesus reaffirmed the ancient commandment when he was questioned by the lawyer: 'You shall love the Lord your God with all your heart, and with all your soul, and with all your mind ... [and] your neighbour as yourself' (Matthew 22.37, 39). Feelings can have a role in our prayers, but only as our wills are under the sovereignty of God.

Sometimes praying can seem just a routine. We read our Bibles and we try to intercede for others, including those who have asked for our prayers and to whom we have ministered, but it all seems stale and empty. Neither our interest nor our emotions are stirred, and we wonder if we should give up trying to pray for a while. That could sound like sensible advice. But if we followed it we would find our spiritual pilgrimage gravely retarded. Loving relationships are not suspended just because we don't happen to feel like them; they aren't suspended on God's side, and they shouldn't be on ours.

Jesus urged his disciples to be persistent in their petitions to the Father and not to be put off by an apparent lack of answers (Luke 18.3–8; see Matthew 15.22–28). A routine of daily prayer can be a demonstration of our faithful desire to return God's love, even when we have little inclination or encouragement to do so. And if we go on trusting him, we shall discover, sometimes long afterwards, that it was through these desert-like times that God drew us closer to himself. Gradually we shall discern his answers to our prayers, and we shall appreciate why spiritual directors teach that praying is as vital to our lives as breathing.

In prayer, then, the Spirit draws us into the divine fellowship of the Holy Trinity by virtue of our baptismal union with Jesus Christ, who is our Advocate and Mediator, our High Priest who 'is able for all time to save those who approach God through him, since he always lives to make intercession for them' (Hebrews 7.25).

Another way of describing it is to see our prayer in the relationship of God over us (the Father), God with us (the Son) and God within us (the Holy Spirit). It is the Spirit *within us* who inspires our desire to draw closer in prayer to the Father who is *over us*, and it is the Son who comes *with us* as we seek the Father.

The Trinitarian nature of our relationship with God is reflected in the wording of liturgical prayers. These are generally addressed to the Father (following our Lord's instruction, 'Pray . . . in this way: "Our Father in heaven . . ."', Matthew 6.9), and end with an ascription such as: 'through Jesus Christ our Lord, who with you and the Holy Spirit lives and reigns for ever and ever'.

The wording of many of these formularies can teach us how the scriptures have inspired Christians in the past to approach God with their hopes and fears, and to express their faith in their prayers. We shouldn't strive to emulate them, for it is best that we address God in our own way; but at least these formularies show how God's word revealed in biblical texts and concepts can assist us to discern our motives when we intercede for others.

Since prayer is such a personal thing, it follows that each of us will approach it in our own way. Sometimes we read formal prayers that express exactly what we want to say, and within which we sense the guiding of the Spirit. At other times we want to pray using our own words, relying on the same Spirit to guide us. Formal prayer can encourage and inspire spontaneous prayer, and spontaneous prayer can help us to appreciate formal prayer. In my experience both kinds can be equally expressive of what we want to say to God personally, and both have their valuable role in the healing ministry.

How, then, does this work out in practice? Here I describe a method of praying that I have found helpful. There are other methods that help different people.

I begin by invoking the Spirit, perhaps saying 'Come, Holy Spirit' a few times, or quietly praying in tongues (the result of involvement with the charismatic renewal). I imagine the Spirit quickening my heart and mind and leading me to Jesus. The use of our imagination in prayer can be helpful provided we have it under control; out of control, it can be a wild distraction!

It may be that in God's presence I become conscious of my unworthiness. Christ died for my sins and, after remembering those faults that trouble my conscience, I make an act of penitence: 'O Lamb of God, who takes away the sins of the world, have mercy upon me.' At all times, and especially before we engage in ministry, it is important that we keep – as my Evangelical friends say – short accounts with God. After that, I move into other kinds of prayer – praise, thanksgiving, intercession – looking to the Father, but conscious I can only approach him because the Holy Spirit unites us to Jesus.

When I am with a suppliant I sometimes imagine stretching out my hand to Christ, and as he takes my hand Christ reaches out and takes the suppliant's hand as well (see Mark 1.41, 9.27; Luke 5.13); then together we approach the Father, believing we are surrounded and indwelt by the Holy Spirit who is guiding and encouraging us.

We naturally hope God will heal them, but we have to trust that the way God wants to do this may not be our way. There may be things in suppliants' lives of which we know nothing but which may hinder gifts of healing. Or there may be situations in which an illness faithfully accepted can be a powerful witness to the grace of God flowing from the cross. We always have to remember that the healing ministry is exercised under the shadow of Calvary as well as before the empty tomb and in the upper room.

I have always felt uncomfortable when I have heard prayers demanding the Lord to heal: that seems to me to be telling God what he ought to do. Equally with exhortations to suppliants to 'claim your healing': that seems to impose on them a heavy but unnecessary burden of responsibility for their healing. Rather, when I pray for a suppliant I try to express our total trust in the Father who loves us, who sent Jesus to be our Saviour and Healer, and who knows what is best for us, and to trust the Holy Spirit to guide me in articulating our hopes in conformity to God's will.

While I am praying, I am often aware of the mental, emotional and psychological processes involved in my response. Naturally my sympathy reaches out to those who ask me to pray for them. I'd love to witness miraculous healings as a result of my intercessions. But personal desires, as I have said, must be submitted to the Lord. In ministry situations such as this we must ask Christ to purify and correct our inner selves so that we can be effective channels of his healing power: that our prayers for others in their sickness and troubles may be, in the famous words of George Herbert, 'God's Breath in man returning to his birth.'

For Discussion

- 'Glory be to the Father, and to the Son, and to the Holy Spirit.' What thoughts or pictures come into your mind as you say these words?
- Do we set limits to what the All Mighty God can do?

6

PRAYING TOGETHER

Chapter Summary

- Ministering together in pairs.
- The roles of the leader and of the assistant.
- Openness to the guiding of the Holy Spirit.
- Listening to suppliants and interceding for them.
- Liturgical and spontaneous prayer.

When team members minister in pairs, one acts as leader and the other as assistant. If one is inexperienced, then he or she acts as the assistant; but when both are experienced, they can exchange roles if they wish with different suppliants, the leader becoming the assistant and vice versa.

Much of what was discussed about intercessory prayer in the last chapter is, of course, applicable when two people are ministering together. There are differences, however, in that each of the pair needs to be alert, not only to the promptings of the Holy Spirit and the needs of the suppliant, but also to their partner's way of responding to God in prayer. It is the difference between singing a solo and taking part in a duet.

Various models of prayer ministry are current today. John Wimber's teaching on inviting the Holy Spirit to come on the suppliant and watching to see what happens to that person is popular, since it focuses the pair's attention on the one for whom they are praying. A development of that is the person centred prayer ministry described by John Leach in a Grove Book of that title. We can learn much from these and other models and then ask God to lead us in the way he wants us to go when we pray with suppliants.

To demonstrate this I shall assume that I am one of a ministering pair and that my assistant is a woman (who in fact is nearly always my wife, Margaret). What I shall also assume is that the circumstances in which we are ministering – time, situation, persons concerned – are ideal. In real life, of course, such circumstances rarely occur. But it does no harm to have a model of some sort in mind, even if we have to depart from it in practice. The model I often use has been drawn from various sources besides those mentioned above. I shall discuss in a later chapter matters such as the laying on of hands, anointing, Communion and following up people who have received ministry.

My assistant and I meet beforehand to pray, invoking the Holy Spirit to equip us with his unity and his gifts. We pray for unity because when we minister in pairs we are manifesting together – if very imperfectly – the love of God in Christ to the suppliants; we pray for spiritual gifts because it is only as the Spirit guides and equips us that we can be the Lord's servants to them.

In the unity and gifts that the Spirit brings, the two of us become a ministering cell within the Body of Christ. Together we are representatives of the community of God's people, acting – or trying to act – in Christ's name. On such occasions I have sometimes had a fresh awareness of what Jesus meant when he promised, 'Where two or three are gathered in my name, I am there among them' (Matthew 18.20).

During our preparatory time together, we try to listen to anything the Lord might reveal to us. Perhaps one of us will be prompted to recall a passage of scripture; the other may be given a word of knowledge. We share these briefly with one another, deciding whether or not they might be helpful to one of the suppliants. This is part of the discerning process: the thoughts of one being tested by the other.

We must beware not to mislead one another unwittingly by our personal anxieties and sympathies. We want to be open to the Holy Spirit, but we cannot assume that every passing idea we have is inspired by him. But if we are reasonably happy with what we hear from one another, we make mental notes of what has been said. When I have been ministering with a woman I have noticed that her perceptions are often different – but not necessarily contradictory – from mine.

Thus prepared, we commence our ministry. The suppliant's approach and our welcome is an outward and visible sign of our coming together in Jesus' name. That doesn't mean, of course, that our suppliants were separated from God before they came to us. What it does mean – to recall the imaginary picture of the last chapter – is that my assistant and I are going to take the suppliant by the hand and bring him or her to Christ. Christ reaches out and embraces the three of us in his Spirit and leads us to the Father.

First we listen to our suppliant, noting their concerns and the way they express themselves. Some of their hopes and fears might be incorporated into our prayers for them later. We try to put ourselves into their situation and to understand what underlies the things they tell us. We only ask a question if it is necessary to clarify what we are to pray for. Sometimes it helps if we enquire, 'And what would you like the Lord to do for you?'

In these prayer ministry encounters, we are not acting as counsellors or spiritual directors. We must be clear about that (see Chapter 8). It is true that certain gifts that enable

Christians to counsel others or to be their spiritual directors have a place in our ministry – especially the charism of discernment – but we are not in those roles here. We are simply the suppliant's intercessors.

As our suppliant speaks or in the few moments afterwards a sentence may come into my mind or a picture into my imagination. It may be something my assistant and I have shared earlier, or it may be completely new. These sort of things do not always happen, and I have to beware of inventing them. It is tempting to make a habit of letting my imagination fabricate 'words of knowledge' or 'inspired pictures' (and acquire a reputation for it!). On the other hand, I am ready to take risks when it seems reasonable to do so, as I know from past experience that such words and pictures can often be very encouraging to suppliants.

As leader, it is my responsibility to initiate the prayers. Sometimes I seem to be guided in what I am to say. But when I haven't any such guidance, I offer a quick arrow prayer and begin speaking slowly and reverently, trusting the Spirit to lead.

I generally address prayer to God the Father, ascribe to him an attribute relevant to the request ('Father God, you give good gifts to your children'; 'Merciful Father, you know our fears and doubts'), and then in a free-wheeling manner let the prayer shape itself. I try to see the suppliant's need in the light of God's grace and allow that to give meaning to what I pray. I may bring into the prayer a scriptural text that comes into my mind, or a phrase used by the suppliant when expressing a fear or hope. Above all, I affirm faith in the Father who loves us, in Christ our Redeemer and Healer, and in the Holy Spirit who renews us as sons and daughters of God. Finally, I offer what I have said in Jesus' name.

I speak clearly and without haste so that the suppliant hears what I am praying. I may pause for a second or two between sentences, trying to discern what I should say next. And I take care not to be too long – certainly not much longer than the words of the previous paragraph. Then I give my assistant an opportunity to add a further prayer.

Her role is slightly different from mine. While she is listening to what I say and observing the suppliant, she is praying silently. When I have finished she may be prompted to add a further prayer, bringing before God an aspect of our suppliant's needs that I haven't mentioned, or she may add further intercessions to supplement mine.

Any scriptural texts, words of encouragement or inspired pictures that my assistant or I may have are usually best shared towards the end of the ministry. It is also advisable to share only one item, or at the most two, so as not to confuse the suppliant. When I do this, I usually preface it by saying: 'I think the Lord has prompted me to tell you . . . (I describe what it is). If it means anything to you, think and pray about it. But if it doesn't, please forget it.'

There are times when I use a set prayer. I do this when I am at a loss to know what to pray, or when I sense the situation requires it – when, for example, time is very short or when I am ministering to a suppliant whom I know is not used to spontaneous prayer and might be distracted by it. It is useful to have a few cards handy with one or two prayers printed on them, such as this from *Common Worship*:

> The almighty Lord, who is a strong tower for all who put
>   their trust in him,
> whom all things in heaven, on earth, and under the earth
>   obey,
> be now and evermore your defence.
> May you believe and trust

> *that the only name under heaven given for health and*
> *salvation*
> *is the name of our Lord Jesus Christ.*

Notice how this prayer is made up of texts from scripture. It recalls the attributes of God as 'a strong tower' (Psalm 61.3; Proverbs 18.10) and of Jesus as the one whom all things 'in heaven, on earth, and under the earth' obey (Philippians 1.10). He is our 'defence' (Psalm 48.3). His is the 'only name' whereby we are saved (Acts 4.12). 'Health and salvation' are closely linked in the New Testament (see Acts 3.16, 4.10, 12). True, as a prayer in the form of a collect for general use, it does not directly invoke the healing gifts of the Holy Spirit, but it resonates with the authority of God's word.

In this and the previous chapter I have described only prayers addressed to God the Father. This is my usual practice. But there are occasions when I feel it is more appropriate to address a prayer to Jesus Christ instead. I do this if I am praying with a child, or if a suppliant shows a particular desire for Jesus to help them. I also adopt this form if I know a suppliant has problems in accepting God as Father; this can be the case with those who in childhood experienced a bad relationship with their parent and who have not yet been healed of the memory of it. As we have seen, many people are brought to faith first through learning about Jesus, so addressing the prayer to him helps them to look to Jesus in hope and faith as their Healer.

If I want to affirm the role of the Holy Spirit and his gifts in ministering, I use an invocation: 'Come, Holy Spirit, we ask you in Jesus' name, and bring your healing gifts (cleansing power . . . conquering strength) . . . that the Father may be glorified . . .'

Whether we address Jesus in our prayer, or invoke the Holy Spirit, we are still within the fellowship of the Holy

Trinity, but we are shaping the prayer we offer so that suppliants can identify themselves with it and are encouraged to look in faith to that Person of the Godhead who in their minds connects with their hopes at that particular time.

One thing I have to watch when I am ministering is that I don't make my prayers so personal that the suppliant and my partner feel excluded from what they are hearing. When praying spontaneously with others, I have to keep in mind that I am speaking for them as well as for myself. Formal prayers, because they are written for general use, avoid that danger.

I end the ministry with the Grace or something similar.

When we have completed our ministry and the suppliants have departed, my assistant and I thank the Lord for what we have been able to do, asking him to confirm what was truly from him in what we have said and done and to overrule any errors we may have made.

There is nothing infallible about our ministry. We can misunderstand our suppliant in such a way that what we have prayed for them has been irrelevant or even insensitive. And, of course, if we need to make amends, we ask the Lord to provide us with an opportunity to do so. But I have to say that I have very rarely met anyone who has been dissatisfied or hurt as a result of this ministry. Most people are grateful that someone has listened to them and prayed for them, even when they have not experienced all they hoped for.

Occasionally, a suppliant may say things that reveal an unwillingness to forgive someone, or resentment of their condition. We wonder for a moment if we should question this. But we are not there to accuse or condemn. Attitudes such as these require a different sort of ministry at another time. So we commend the suppliant to the love of the Father and trust that the Holy Spirit will lead them to where the light of Christ will shine into their darkness.

For Discussion

- Do you prefer to pray using your own thoughts and words spontaneously, or using an appropriate book of prayers?
- What helps you listen to God's voice?

7

Team Meetings

Chapter Summary

- The team and its leader.
- Membership.
- Accountable to the pastoral leadership of a congregation.
- Agenda for meetings, including: intercessory prayer for the sick, ongoing teaching, supporting and ministering to one another.
- Links with Christians in the caring professions.

The parish priest is usually the team leader, at least to begin with. If leadership is delegated to someone else, then they should report to the priest regularly. What the team is being trained for is an important expression of the pastoral care of the congregation, for which the priest is ultimately responsible under the bishop. The team therefore exercises its ministry under his authority. When he is not leading the team, a wise priest will make a point of attending its meetings from time to time to keep in touch.

For this reason policy decisions concerning the team's ministry should have the priest's consent. The team may put forward certain suggestions about which the priest may feel he or she should first consult the parochial church council or even the diocesan bishop. As far as the rest of the congregation is concerned, an occasional report on the team's work to the parochial church council gives the council a chance to discuss it.

Membership has to be reviewed at times. Individuals begin to drop out of the team. They move away from the area, or they believe the Lord is calling them to undertake other work. Then the team has to pray and look for new recruits.

Now and then a member may cease to attend meetings without offering an apology or an explanation. To avoid embarrassment when this situation arises, the team should have a rule, which is understood by everyone who joins, that if any of them ceases to attend meetings without good reasons for, say, six months, they will be asked if they wish to continue their membership. They need to realize that the team is not a casual club to which people come and go as they wish; it is an arm of the Church's mission involving the health and welfare of the congregation (and perhaps others), and membership has to be a personal and disciplined commitment. If such a rule is adopted when the team is formed, it will make it easier for the leader to approach persistent absentees later.

Team meetings include:

Intercessory prayer. Since the team's ministry is founded on prayer, the practice of praying is high on its agenda. This includes prayer for each other, and for individuals who have received ministry or who are known to be sick or troubled; for those in the caring professions; and for those looking after ailing relatives or friends. Thanksgivings for the past and prayers for the future are also appropriate. Some teams will want to include songs of praise. My *Healed, Restored, Forgiven* contains examples of prayers for a variety of situations in which team members and suppliants may find themselves – alone, at meetings, and before and after services.

Teaching. As we saw in the previous chapter, ongoing training helps to keep members fresh in their understanding of and hopes about their ministry. Courses are worth repeating every two or three years with existing members as well as new ones. What has been learned before often has a new relevance after a few years' ministering to people. Many of the questions that arise as the team becomes more experienced in their ministry are discussed in *A Time to Heal*.

A visit to other churches for their team meetings or healing services broadens horizons, as do return visits. These exchanges need not be limited to Anglicans. It is often enlightening to find out how clergy and teams in other denominations are exercising the ministry in their own traditions, from Roman Catholic healing Masses to Pentecostal evangelistic rallies.

The purpose of all training is that members of the group may exercise the gift of discernment when they listen to suppliants and be open to the leading of the Holy Spirit when they minister in prayer.

Ministering in pairs. Ministering in pairs itself is a learning experience. Indeed, I think it is difficult for anyone to embark on this ministry without first working alongside a more experienced colleague. Nearly everything I have learned has come through sharing in the ministry of others. Afterwards I often asked them, 'Why did you say this?' and, 'Why did you do that?'

Books on the ministry recommend that pairs should, if possible, be made up of a man and a woman. I endorse that, but I want to add a word of warning. Years ago I was at a conference on the ministry of healing at a Christian residential centre. Among the guests were a middle-aged clergyman and a woman. I noticed that they walked about with their arms affectionately round one another, and I assumed that they were married and enjoying a kind of second honeymoon.

One day when I was talking to them I happened to remark, 'It's good that you and your wife were able to come together on this conference.' It was immediately evident that my comment embarrassed them. They instinctively drew slightly apart, and the clergyman hesitatingly replied: 'Oh, we're not married. We minister together in the parish. You see, my wife is not interested in this sort of thing.' I noticed that they avoided me for the rest of the week.

When he gave lectures on what he called Clinical Theology (Christian counselling) to the clergy in the diocese where I served, Dr Frank Lake warned us to be careful if we ministered together regularly with a member of the opposite sex. Unless they are watchful, he said, men and women in this situation can become emotionally attracted to one another, particularly after being jointly involved in the troubles of their suppliants. That can have unhappy consequences if they have a wife and a husband; they become, in his well-known phrase, 'a gruesome twosome'.

Planning. If there is a healing service in the near future, the priest with the team plans the arrangements in consultation with the musicians and sidespersons and others involved. At their next meeting after the service they review how it went and make arrangements for any follow-up of individuals that may be necessary. Further suggestions are made about this in Chapters 9 and 10.

The team's ministry is not confined to healing services,

however. Members who visit the sick or who encounter people with particular troubles may be asked to pray with them. In some parishes a team pair is on duty after the Sunday services in a quiet corner of the church for anyone who comes seeking ministry for a personal matter.

Sharing. Some members of these teams can come under a good deal of pressure as they seek to help others in their anxieties and suffering, and it is important that they should receive pastoral care themselves and know that they are supported. The team meeting is often an opportunity for this, and so there should be time for members to share their own concerns and to discuss problems that they are encountering. It is during these discussions that matters of confidentiality and boundaries crop up, and they need to be handled with care (see Chapter 8). But, of course, members are free to seek advice elsewhere if they wish.

Written notes. Provided team members are not involved in too many cases and their corporate memory is reliable, there is no need for notes to be made. But if the ministry expands to such an extent that it is difficult to remember the decisions that have been made and the suppliants who require ongoing attention, then notes may be necessary in the interests of pastoral efficiency. They should be written in such a way that, if others read them, they do not reveal anything personal. They should be shredded when they are no longer needed.

The team and the congregation. Besides their occasional reports to the church council, the team ought to review its relationship with the rest of the congregation from time to time. Groups drawn together by a common task can tend to give an impression of exclusiveness. Most team members don't want to give this impression, but they should be aware that others might feel it. They can help to dispel this impression by taking part in other activities in the church fellowship. Their ministry is more welcomed and appreciated if they are seen to be as committed to the congregation as they are to the team. Having said that, however, occasional social gatherings for the team help to build up its esprit de corps.

The key to the healing ministry, as in all ministries, is that it is inspired by the love of God. Where the team is concerned, this manifests itself in a humble willingness to be of service to others, a sensitive understanding of the pastoral responsibilities for which the priest is ordained, and a prayerful loyalty to one another.

For Discussion

- If, during a team meeting, you felt that someone was being given unwise advice, how would you deal with the situation?
- Does the team ever discuss the problems faced by members of the congregation, and others who have disabilities (mobility, hearing, etc.) and what they should do about them?

8

CONFIDENTIALITY AND BOUNDARIES

Chapter Summary

- Importance of observing rules of confidentiality.
- Knowing when and how to set boundaries to the team's ministry.
- A congregation's trust in the ministry of the team.
- Personal relationships between team members and their suppliants.
- The value of advisers from the caring professions.

When I was a young priest, the post-ordination tutor who lectured us on how to hear confessions (or to preside at the ministry of reconciliation, as it is called these days) emphasized the importance of 'the seal'. We were told that we must never, under any circumstances, reveal to anyone what we heard when a penitent made their confession. Only if a penitent gives permission were we to raise with them afterwards any matter they had mentioned in the confessional.

The reason is obvious. Privacy and protection are essential if penitents are to be free to make a genuine confession. The seal is their guarantee that confidentiality will be observed. Sins are confessed primarily to God; as priests, we were told, we hear confessions only as representatives of the Body of Christ. A truly penitent sinner is reconciled both to God through the saving grace of Jesus and to his Church to which they are joined by baptism.

The ministry of reconciliation only concerns a member of the healing prayer team if a suppliant is advised to make their confession as a step towards their healing – and in any case it is more likely such advice will be given by the priest rather than by a member of the team. But the code of confidentiality is just as important in all the team's ministry with suppliants, and it should be strictly observed.

People are entitled to expect that what they say to members of the team will be treated as confidential. This gives them the freedom to not hold anything back if they have a burden they wish to share. Should they have any reason to suspect that information about them will become the topic of parish gossip, trust in the team will immediately be destroyed – not only the suppliant's but also of those who hear the gossip.

It may be necessary for team members to set limits on the degree of confidentiality if, for example, a suppliant reveals they have a complex personal problem that team members feel they are not competent or trained to handle. In that case they have to explain this to the suppliant and ask if he or she would like them to refer the matter to the priest or to an authorized counsellor. If the suppliant refuses, then the team member must respect that decision and end the ministry with a prayer.

Confidentiality extends to the team's family and friends. When we get home after a healing service or a ministry session we may feel an urge to describe what we have been doing. Or when we've listened to a troubled teenager pouring out their problems involving their parents, we may feel we ought to go and talk to the parents to help them see their teenager's point of view. But such actions would be a breach of confidentiality.

I want to stress, however, that it is quite in order for us to ask a suppliant if we can share what they have told us with the priest or the team in order to get further advice. They may agree to this if they think it will help them and us. Discussing suppliants' problems with the team helps members to share any burdens of responsibility they may feel, and also provides the team with an opportunity to learn more about their ministry.

Sharing cases with the team in this way has another advantage. Very occasionally a deeply disturbed suppliant will go from one member of the team to another – not primarily to listen to advice or to receive prayer, but to engage the attention of others without the discomfort of facing their own problems. By sharing any experience of this kind, team members are alerted to the possibility that they are being manipulated by that particular suppliant.

The boundaries of confidentiality can be overstepped quite unintentionally during times of prayer in church services or elsewhere. Naturally we want to encourage the congregation to pray for suppliants, and in cases where the illnesses and troubles of individuals are known to the congregation it is entirely proper that we should do so. But when we are praying publicly for someone who has given us information that is confidential, then we must be careful that we don't say anything in our prayers that reveals their identity.

This is a special danger in smaller churches where everyone knows one another. For example, we might during the general intercessions invite the congregation to pray for a school teacher who has to decide whether or not to resign from her job because she has been told she has an incurable illness. It could be that there is only one woman in that congregation who fits that description and so, of course, all those who hear the request immediately guess who it is. If the teacher wanted her problem to be kept confidential for the time being, that could be very embarrassing for her, even hurtful.

In the same way we must not use confidential information about individuals as illustrations in sermons or training sessions without their permission. It is not uncommon for those of us who are asked to give talks on the healing ministry to draw on our experiences in order to add interest to what we are saying. But if we want to use a certain case for this purpose, we must make sure we disguise the names and the circumstances in such a way that the suppliant concerned can never be identified. Even so, I would strongly advise that such illustrations are not used within a congregation or a group of churches where there may be listeners who will recognize the person we are telling them about in spite of the disguises.

Drawing the lines of the boundaries in personal relationships can sometimes be difficult. Inevitably some of those who ask us to pray for them will be personal friends or acquaintances. Normally this should not cause any difficulty; after all, they approach us voluntarily. It is unlikely that they will reveal anything that we don't know already or that will embarrass our relationship. Indeed, it is a privilege when friends and acquaintances seek our ministry in this way. Yet we must be careful not to react if they tell us something about their situation that comes as a complete surprise to us.

Relationships both within the team ministry and with our suppliants also require sagacious boundaries. When an individual shares with us the more intimate details of their life, we would be less than human if there were occasions when we were not moved with a deep sympathy for them.

Emotional responses like this within ourselves need to be recognized and controlled; we ought to be self-aware enough to be able to deal with them as they arise.

I am not suggesting that we cannot form warm relationships with other people where it is appropriate to do so within the bounds of normal Christian behaviour. But what I described as a 'gruesome twosome' in the previous chapter can also apply in the relationship of a team member with a suppliant. Particularly vulnerable are those men and women whose marriages are going through a difficult time, and individuals who are lonely and depressed. Such people may become deeply attached to those who listen sympathetically to them and pray for them. Keeping a proper emotional and psychological distance from one another, yet also maintaining a unity in the Holy Spirit, can be a testing business. Unless we are watchful, the devil has a subtle way of twisting our relationships so that they become injurious, not healing.

Then there are the boundaries that the team members have to accept for themselves. We should not engage in ministries that lead us beyond the skills with which we have been gifted or those for which we have not been trained and authorized. Nor are we permitted to attempt any kind of deliverance ministry beyond a simple prayer for protection from evil. At all times we are to minister under the direction of the pastoral leadership of our church, which in most places will be the team leader or the priest.

Where a suppliant needs further help beyond what we or the team can provide, we should advise them about this but take no steps without their consent. They should be informed of the nature of this help and probably given time to go away and think about it. That avoids placing them in a position where they have to make a decision on the spur of the moment. We must resist every tendency to try and control our suppliants – a temptation faced by any of us who happens to think we know what is good for someone else!

A special warning needs to be given to the team about ministering to children and young people. Current legislation is strict about this, and it is advisable that members who are drawn into this kind of ministry receive proper clearance for it.

One of the reasons why a team can benefit from having advisers is that they can help us to recognize our boundaries. We must not trespass in matters that are the responsibility of those in the caring professions. But at times it is helpful to seek advice from them informally. In my experience most of them are willing to help, provided they are not being asked to breach their own rules of confidentiality and they are satisfied we are acting in a responsible manner.

Finally, we have to observe a proper boundary between ourselves and those to whom we have ministered in the follow-up. In some cases it might be necessary to see a certain suppliant after we have prayed with them to see how they are getting on. But in our eagerness to hear whether or not our ministry has been a 'success' (if we fall into the trap of regarding ourselves in that way) we must never, never, try to persuade them to say that they feel better, or that they have been healed. It is up to them to decide when and where to claim such things, and to give the glory not to us, but to God.

For Discussion

- If you wanted the team to pray for someone without revealing who that person was, how would you do this?
- What would you look for in the person with whom you feel you could share confidential matters about yourself?

9

PREPARATIONS FOR
A HEALING SERVICE

Chapter Summary

- Preparing for a healing service.
- Decisions about the kind of service within which the healing ministry is offered.
- Planning the content of the service with all those involved.
- Practical arrangements for the team in church.
- Prayer before the service.

When the team are sufficiently trained, preparations are made for them to minister in a public service for the first time. Some weeks beforehand the vicar has to decide what kind of a service this is to be. A Eucharist? A traditional evening service? An informal service of prayer and praise? Or a service of thanksgiving for the ministry of healing from *Common Worship*?

Whatever form the service takes, the team's role is much the same. However, to explain these preparations I will imagine I am the vicar of the church in which it is being arranged.

I have decided, in consultation with the team and the parochial church council, that I will preside at a *Common*

Worship Eucharist and that the team will minister at it in pairs. I begin by choosing the scripture readings, if those provided for the day in the lectionary are not appropriate. As I will be the preacher, I need to give myself time to think and pray about the sermon, especially as this is the first time many in the congregation will have been to such a service.

My next step is to meet the others who will be involved. I discuss the theme of the service and the arrangements with the director of music and with his or her help choose the hymns, songs and any other music that is required. I then brief the choir or the music group, again explaining the theme of the service and the arrangements being made for it. I emphasize firmly that during the time suppliants are receiving ministry they are to play or sing quietly, with the public address system turned low; I point out to them that it is difficult for the team and their suppliants to hear one another if the organ is being played fortissimo and songs are being belted out to the accompaniment of drums and cymbals! I also meet the churchwardens and sidespersons and discuss the arrangements for the service with them.

In the meantime I have been drawing up an outline of the service. At a Eucharist there are two points at which the kind of ministry we are planning can be offered.

The first is to put the ministry immediately after the Confession and Absolution:

Preliminary rites (Introduction, Collect, etc.)
The Ministry of the Word
The Sermon
The Intercessions
The Confession and Absolution
The Ministry of Prayer with the Laying on of Hands
The Peace
The Eucharistic Prayer, etc.

The Communion
Concluding rites

The logic behind this pattern is that the Ministry of the Word is intended to teach us and to stir our faith in preparation for what follows. In the intercessions we remember those in need and especially the sick who cannot be present; then we join in the corporate confession of sin and receive the assurance of God's forgiveness – an important element in the healing ministry for all of us. From this we move into the Ministry of Prayer with the Laying on of Hands. When that finishes everyone joins in exchanging the Peace with one another. The climax of the service is the Eucharistic Prayer and the Communion, our great thanksgiving to God for his mercy and grace.

This liturgical pattern is followed when individuals and groups are receiving a blessing or being commissioned during a Eucharist – e.g. at a wedding, a baptism, a confirmation or an ordination.

However, it only works well when the congregation is small and there are few suppliants. With a large number the gap between the Absolution and the Peace is prolonged and it is not easy for a congregation to concentrate all that time unless they are very disciplined worshippers. So, as I am expecting a large congregation, I opt for an alternative pattern:

Preliminary rites (Introduction, Collect, etc.)
The Confession and Absolution, either here or after the Intercessions
The Ministry of the Word
The Sermon
The Intercessions
The Peace

The Eucharistic Prayer, etc.
The Communion
The Ministry of Prayer with the Laying on of Hands
Concluding rites

The advantage of this alternative pattern is that if the ministry to individuals goes on longer than is reasonable, I will be able as president to lead the congregation through the rest of the service, hoping the team will have finished their ministering by the time we get to the Dismissal.

With the plan of the service settled, I meet the team in church a few days beforehand to work out the practical details. There are various places where the team can pray with individuals during a service, but much depends on the layout of the interior of the church.

A simple way is for Prayer with the Laying on of Hands to be offered at the communion rail. Suppliants stand or kneel as the members of the team, working in pairs, move from one to the next, rather as when the bread and the wine are distributed. This is a suitable arrangement if only prayers (and anointing) are administered in a formal manner with set prayers. Its disadvantage is that if suppliants want to give the team information about their needs, and questions are asked, others standing or kneeling next to them can overhear what is being said, which may be inhibiting.

To avoid this problem, the team pairs stand in the sanctuary or the chancel – if there are three pairs, one at each side and one in the middle – so that suppliants can come to them individually. In these positions there is less chance of what is said being overheard.

If a side chapel is available, chairs can be arranged in different corners and the team can minister to their suppliants sitting. This provides a degree of privacy and it is easier for the pairs and their suppliants to hear one another.

In churches that are fairly spacious, chairs can also be set up in different places ('stations') in the aisles or at the back. This is how we decide to operate, but I have to warn the team that when they are sitting they should take care suppliants don't become comfortable in their chairs and use the opportunity for a lengthy chat!

At the services on the previous Sunday I inform the congregation what is to take place. Reminding them of what I have taught them about the healing ministry, I explain carefully what those who are to receive ministry will be expected to do. I say that I am ready to discuss it with anyone who wants further help in making up their minds, adding that I am willing to make other arrangements for individuals who do not wish to receive this ministry in public.

I stress that the healing ministry is not solely something the team does; it is a ministry of the whole congregation, and their prayers for suppliants are just as important as those offered by the team. If they see people coming and going for ministry, that is a chance to pray for them individually.

Publicity requires some care. I do not want this first service to be advertised so widely that we find many coming to church who are not members of the congregation. A sensationalized report in the local newspaper ('Healings Expected in Parish Church!') will send the wrong sort of messages into the neighbourhood. Maybe one day we shall be able to welcome anyone who wants to come, but a healing service planned as part of the Church's mission in the parish is not what we can handle at this stage. Initially we are offering the ministry to the members of our own congregation and any relatives or friends they bring along with them.

So the Sunday for the service arrives. I meet the team an hour before it begins, if possible in a place where we will not be disturbed. We briefly go over the arrangements once more, including who will pair with whom, and then spend time praying for those who are coming to the service. We do this methodically, naming those who are actively involved – the president, preacher, musicians, sidespersons, and so on – and then the congregation, mentioning any who have told us they are going to come forward for ministry.

The congregation, of course, will have been aware for some time that a team has been training for this. Many know the members of the team personally. But there will be others who do not, so I have arranged for the team to wear badges with their names printed boldly on them.

At this point I will discard my role as an imaginary vicar and add a final comment.

For many years now I have belonged to a church where there are other clergy; this has meant that at healing services I have been free to act as a member of the team and to meet with them before the service. I've gone with them into the church without having to check that the sidespersons have given out the right books or been informed that the public address system is not working (the kind of emergencies that all too frequently harass a clergyman in the minutes before the worship begins!).

I realize therefore that this preparatory meeting with the team may not be possible for many clergy. They may have to leave the team to be responsible for its own devotions before a service. But even if the priest only has time to visit them briefly beforehand, that can be an encouragement in these early stages of the team's development.

In the next chapter we will discuss the service and the follow-up, continuing in my imaginary vicar's role.

For Discussion

- What single passage from the following parts of the Bible would you choose to be read at a service of prayer for healing: (1) the Psalms; (2) the Old Testament; (3) the Gospels; (4) the rest of the New Testament?

- A friend says to you, 'I'd love to ask for prayer at the next healing service, but I don't want to have to get up and walk forward in front of everybody.' How would you reply?

10

MINISTRY DURING A SERVICE

Chapter Summary

- Ministry to suppliants during a service.
- Watchfulness by the one who presides.
- Personal testimonies.
- Encouraging suppliants to accept ministry.
- The after-service conversations.
- Warning of possibility of a spiritual backlash.

The Eucharist from *Common Worship* begins in the usual way. The prayer ministry team members are seated at the ends of the rows of seats so that they can get in and out without having to push past others. During the introductory remarks I remind the congregation of what I told them the previous Sunday. For the benefit of any who weren't there, I quickly explain how the ministry is to be offered, pointing out the stations round the church where the pairs of ministers will be sitting, and explaining that the sidespersons will direct individuals who come forward for prayer. I also remind the congregation that their prayers during the time of ministry are as important as those offered by the team.

As it happened a man belonging to the congregation had experienced a measure of healing after he had been prayed for at another church recently while he was on holiday with his family, and I had invited him to give a testimony about it. We had met the previous day to make notes and rehearse what he was going to say; I was anxious that he should be brief without omitting important details. He came forward and did this at a pre-arranged point during my sermon, so that his testimony became one of my illustrations.

I had originally planned to ask different members of the team to read the scriptures and to lead the intercessions, but changed my mind. I decided it would be better to use other people. That would leave the team free to concentrate on their own role in the service.

I use Eucharistic Prayer C as that is one with which the congregation are most familiar. I include in it one of the proper prefaces for general use on occasions like this:

> *It is right to give you thanks*
> *in sickness and in health,*
> *in suffering and in joy,*
> *through Christ our Saviour and Redeemer,*
> *who as the Good Samaritan*
> *tends the wounds of body and spirit.*
> *He stands by us and pours out for our healing*
> *the oil of consolation and the wine of renewed hope,*
> *turning the darkness of our pain*
> *into the dawning light of his kingdom.*

After everyone has received Communion, the members of the team stand before me while I offer a prayer for them, and they disperse to their stations. I then invite those who wish to receive ministry to come forward.

Two women had told me the previous week that they would like to receive prayer at this service, so I had asked them to get out of their seats as soon as they heard me make the invitation. I had explained to them that when invitations are made like this in church, there is often an awkward pause as no one wants to make the first move; but when one or two come forward, it encourages others to do the same. I am relieved to see this is what happens. The two women had no sooner sat down at two of the stations than several in the congregation were indicating to the sidespersons that they wished to come forward as well.

As the numbers of suppliants increase I am tempted to speed things up by praying with a few of them myself, but I know this would be inadvisable. It is a psychological fact that a crowd of people soon lose their sense of togetherness once the one who is presiding over them is distracted. We see this happen at a public meeting when the chairperson is called away and people begin chatting to their neighbours. It is not always easy to call them to order again!

A mixture of criticism and amusement spread in the Church of England when it was discovered that in the new service books the familiar names of those who lead worship had been changed from 'Priest' or 'Minister' to 'President'. What would Anglicans in the USA make of this? was one comment I heard. But the change was a reminder that the job of the one who leads the liturgy, ordained or lay, is to preside.

I stand in a position where I can watch over the proceedings and see the team ministering to people. I beckon the sidespersons if they overlook someone wanting to go forward. Fortunately the musicians have remembered my request and are playing quietly. As the ministry takes longer than I expected, I lead the congregation in one or two responsorial prayers during a break in the music.

In the meantime I notice that one of teams have placed their chairs at such an angle that the suppliant can look past them to the congregation beyond. This is obviously a distraction for the woman suppliant; as the team are praying for her, I see that her eyes are wandering anxiously over the

church, perhaps wondering what the rest of the congregation are thinking of her. I must tell the team to arrange their
chairs in future so that their suppliants have their backs to
the congregation.

Then I notice something else. The sidespersons are
allowing little queues to form as suppliants wait for their
turn at the stations. That's unfortunate. Queues can be a
disturbing element; they are reminders of the check-outs in
the supermarket where people are in a hurry and impatient
to be served. I make a mental note to tell the sidespersons to
let the suppliants stay in their places until one of the stations
is free. In some churches it is possible for the suppliants,
having received Communion, to sit in the choir stalls or the
front pews reserved for them.

At last the prayer ministry finishes and I am able to
continue the service. Just before the dismissal, however,
I announce that coffee is being served at the back of the
church and that if anyone wishes to see me or a member of
the team we will be there.

We collect our cups and stand around in groups chatting.
The team members and I find ourselves talking to some of
the suppliants but, bearing in mind our rule of confidentiality, we do not say anything about what we have prayed
with them unless they do so first.

Shortly after the service I meet the team to review what
happened and discuss how these could be improved next
time. I mention the things I have observed that need
correcting. Then I find out if there is anyone who has asked
for further ministry or who would welcome an opportunity for a further talk with us. One of the team says she is
concerned about a personal matter that arose as she was
ministering to someone: I suggest she discusses it with me
privately afterwards.

Some churches find that to include a healing ministry

within the context of a Eucharist makes the service too long. Also, it is not always appropriate in churches when a proportion of those who attend are not communicants. It may be better to offer the healing ministry during Evening Prayer or in a more informal service. This helps to familiarize everybody with this ministry and to accept it as part of the normal routine of Sunday worship. Then, once it has become established, it is not difficult to transfer it to a Eucharist, if it is felt desirable to do so. (I have printed suggested texts for different kinds of services in *Healed, Restored, Forgiven*, pages 53–71.)

One further thing needs to be said about our involvement as a team with healing services. It is not uncommon to experience an emotional or spiritual backlash after we have been ministering. When we have been invoking the name of Jesus on behalf of others and relying on the gifts of the Holy Spirit, it is one of the devil's tactics to try and undermine our faith by tempting us to ungodly attitudes and behaviour afterwards. For example, we might find ourselves suddenly having a row with another member of the team, or getting upset about a trivial matter at home.

Watchfulness is a necessary defence against these attacks. But we should not be discouraged by them. By his cross Christ defeated all the powers of the enemy and that victory can be ours when we seek to be reconciled with one another. We call on the Lord by renewing our baptismal renunciation of sin and evil, and ask that these signs of our weakness keep us humble and dependent on his strength. That, after all, is the spiritual springboard of all ministries. 'I am among you as one who serves' (Luke 22.27).

For Discussion

- You are the leader of a pair ministering to an individual who is taking so long to explain their need that the service is being delayed. What would you do?

- The person you are praying with suddenly sinks to the floor and lies still with their eyes shut. What would you do?

11

SACRAMENTAL MINISTRIES

Chapter Summary

- Sacraments and sacramentals in the Church's healing ministry.
- Taking Communion to the sick at home or in hospital.
- Lists of requirements for this.
- Forms of service.
- Administering Communion, anointing and the laying on of hands.

Since healing means wholeness in its fullest sense, then all the sacraments and sacramental signs of the Church are part of the healing ministry. However, healing prayer teams are only likely to be involved in two of these: Holy Communion and Anointing. In this chapter we shall look at the practical matters concerning these.

In the Church of England lay people have to be authorized by the bishop if they are to administer the Sacrament to communicants at a Eucharist in church and take Communion to the sick. Most dioceses make it a condition that candidates go through a course of training before they are given permission to do this. If any members of the team are to become eucharistic ministers, as they are sometimes called, they should be authorized in the usual way. Then they will be able to take Communion to those who are sick at home or housebound, or in hospital or nursing homes.

Different parishes have their own customs for this. What I shall describe is the procedure most churches follow when they take the Sacrament to communicants in their own homes; it may have to be modified if Communion is taken elsewhere.

Communion is taken to the sick in one of two ways. The first is when the Eucharist is celebrated in the presence of the sick person in their home. *Common Worship* makes provision for this. Since it is only done by a priest or bishop, it lies outside the team's responsibility, though the clergy may invite a team member to accompany them on such occasions.

The second is when the Sacrament is taken from the church to the sick. The consecrated bread and wine (or more commonly just the bread) are reserved in a small safe (an aumbry) in the church or in the vestry; it is usually renewed each week at one of the Eucharistic celebrations.

The most convenient method of reserving the bread is by consecrating specially made wafers. Small pieces from an ordinary loaf go hard and stale very quickly, whereas wafers (hosts) can be kept in airtight containers for many weeks without deteriorating. The wine is kept in a small flask.

In some churches only the bread is reserved and Communion given in one kind. In others Communion is given by intinction; that is, after it has been consecrated, the bread is moistened with a drop of the wine and allowed to dry before being reserved. The advantages of this method are that the eucharistic minister does not have to carry a flask of wine and a chalice to the house of the sick person, and the communicant is able to receive both the bread and the wine together in the host (which is usually more acceptable for those Anglicans who are not used to receiving Communion in one kind).

It is also possible to take the Sacrament straight to the sick at home after a Eucharist in church. For this the practical arrangements are the same as when the reserved Sacrament is used.

The eucharistic minister requires:

A pyx (a small box) containing the bread and, if possible, a paten (a small plate) from which to administer it. If the wine is taken in a flask, a chalice will also be required. Most churches have sick Communion sets which contain these vessels in a carrying case.

A corporal (a white cloth about 15 inches square).

A purificator (a smaller cloth for drying the chalice, unless tissues are used).

A Bible.

Books or cards containing the words of the prayers that are to be used (large print ones if the patient has poor eyesight). Church House Publishing have produced a handy card with prayers printed on it from *Common Worship* for giving Communion at home or in hospital. These cards can also be used when a Eucharist is celebrated.

Holy oil, if the patient is to be anointed.

If the eucharistic minister wears a badge of office when administering the sacrament at church services, this can be taken and put on in the house.

Those caring for the sick person should be asked to prepare, if possible:

A table with a cloth spread on it.

A small jug of water and a small basin.

A clean handkerchief or a box of tissues.

One or two lighted candles and a vase of flowers on the table help to create a peaceful atmosphere. A cross or crucifix give a sense of the room being converted into a chapel for the occasion, though obviously it is not always possible for these to be provided.

Enquiries should be made beforehand to find out if any of the sick person's relatives or friends are to receive Communion. This will determine how many breads and how much wine is required. It is not customary for ministers to receive Communion themselves at these services, though there is no reason why they should not do so.

If two members of the team go together, this is often welcomed by patients. They help to create a sense of the patient being part of the wider congregation. As usual, one acts as leader and the other as assistant.

On arriving at the house, the minister asks the patient if prayer is needed for anything special. If this is the first time the patient has received Communion at home, it may be necessary to explain how the service is to be conducted and how the Sacrament is to be administered. This needs to be done without any fuss; the patient should be helped to feel relaxed and not concerned about 'doing the wrong thing'.

The minister then spreads the corporal out on the table and places the paten (and the chalice) on it and the bread on the paten (and pours the wine into the chalice). After a brief period of silence for recollection, the minister begins the service, which consists of the following:

Prayer of Preparation ('Almighty God, to whom all hearts are open')

Confession
Absolution
Collect
One or more readings from Scripture, including a Gospel
Intercessions
Laying on of hands with Prayer (and Anointing, if previously arranged)
The Peace
Lord's Prayer
Administration of the Sacrament
Final Prayer
Grace or Blessing

If the patient is seriously ill, many of these items can be omitted; at least the Confession, the Absolution, the Lord's Prayer, the Final Prayer and the Grace or Blessing should be said.

After the service the minister performs the ablutions: consumes any of the bread and wine that remain, rinses the paten and the chalice with water, dries them with the purificator or tissues, and packs them away. If anointing has been administered, fingers also need to be cleansed.

General conversation is best left until after the service. Ministers should not remain too long if the patient is weak and tired. Otherwise the occasion can be treated as a normal pastoral visit.

Taking Communion to persons in hospitals or care homes calls for much flexibility. Preparations in such places vary considerably. In some hospitals special provision is made for a patient to receive Communion, but not everywhere. Generally speaking, it is best for the official chaplain, if there is one, to administer the Sacrament, as they will have made their own arrangements with the staff and patients.

In any case, as a matter of courtesy, chaplains should be informed if a patient who is nominally under their care receives Communion from someone else.

The fact that Communion has been taken to the sick should be noted later in the church's service register.

For anointing in church or elsewhere the procedure is much the same. Olive oil is used, sometimes with a perfume added, though this is not necessary. It is blessed by a bishop or a priest. In many dioceses the bishop presides at a Eucharist to which his clergy bring their oils to be blessed by him for use during the year. Traditionally these services take place during Holy Week.

The holy oil can be administered straight from the small bottle that contains it. This method can be rather messy unless care is taken not to use too much oil (Psalm 133.2 comes to mind!). Also the bottles, being so small, can easily be knocked over. Instead, ecclesiastical shops sell small circular silver-plated boxes with screw tops which are more convenient. The box is filled with some absorbent material like cotton wool and the holy oil poured into it. The minister dips his or her thumb or middle finger (I generally use the latter) into the box and makes the mark of a small cross on the forehead of the suppliant, saying a prayer such as this from *Common Worship*:

> *N., I anoint you in the name of God who gives you life.*
> *Receive Christ's forgiveness, his healing and his love.*
> *May the Father of our Lord Jesus Christ*
> *grant you the riches of his grace,*
> *his wholeness and his peace. Amen.*

When ministering the laying on of hands to someone in a bed, it is sufficient to hold the patient's hand when praying, or to gently place a hand on his or her shoulder.

For Discussion

- How would you feel – if you were a housebound invalid – if Communion was brought to you at home from the church by an authorized lay person whom you didn't like very much?
- In the case of a long-term illness, how frequently should the suppliant be anointed?

12

FURTHER DEVELOPMENTS

Chapter Summary

- Evolution of a congregation's healing ministry.
- Ministers in pairs pray with individuals after services.
- Teams assist in training programmes elsewhere.
- Individuals feel called to undertake further training in counselling.
- Groups, communities and homes of healing.

Healing prayer teams may develop in different ways. In some churches, where healing services have been established for a few years, ministry to individuals is offered at all the Sunday services on a regular monthly or two-monthly basis. On these days no special attempt is made to focus on the healing ministry; the services are celebrated much as usual and suppliants receive prayer and the laying on of hands without detailed explanations and instructions. The ministry has become an accepted part of the congregation's worship and life.

Another development, mentioned earlier, is to offer this ministry after the Sunday services for individuals who feel they need personal prayer support at that time. The team pairs, working on a rota that appears on the same service sheet as the names of the sidespersons and scripture readers, sit in a quiet corner of the church when the service has finished and wait for suppliants to approach them informally. I have been a member of such a pair on a once-a-month rota for several years, and on average someone has come to us for prayer about one out of every two Sundays I've been on duty.

Not everyone asks for prayer for healing. They come for all sorts of reasons: a schoolgirl anxious about a forthcoming examination; a youth concerned about his parents' pending divorce; a mother worried about a daughter on drugs; a man unhappy at work; an elderly person going to hospital for the first time; and so on. I think this kind of ministry is just as valued as that offered in the formal healing services.

Do these developments mean that we should expect formal services for healing to disappear in time? I don't think so. Occasional healing services enable the Church to demonstrate publicly that we are trying to fulfil the ministry of Christ the Healer, and that healing is a manifestation of the Kingdom that he came to proclaim. The first sentence in the report *A Time to Heal* reads: 'The healing ministry is one of the greatest opportunities the Church has today for sharing the Gospel' (page xiii). It is an aspect of this ministry that the Church must not forget.

Then there are developments outside the parish. Such is the interest in the healing ministry these days that a parochial team known to be experienced in it may get called on to share their knowledge with others.

They may be invited to lead teaching courses in other churches – just as a visiting team helped the vicar to establish the ministry in my imaginary parish in Chapter 2. At a big diocesan gathering I attended shortly after *A Time to Heal* was published, members of five teams spoke on the way in which they exercised their ministry in their own parishes. It was an impressive act of witness – all the more so (in Anglican circles, at least) because it was entirely led by the laity.

Members of the team may also be asked to speak on the healing ministry at Christian centres and national gatherings. Conference centres frequently include the healing ministry in their programmes and invite members of a parish team to lead it; national gatherings such as Spring Harvest and New Wine do the same. These conferences often end with a service at which the team takes part by praying with suppliants.

In time one or two members of the team may feel the Lord is calling them to develop their personal ministries in different ways. Individuals begin to realize that they are often being approached by suppliants with similar problems, who seem to regard them as being more gifted to help them than others in the team. This form of specialization in the charisms is not uncommon. The Lord uses whatever natural abilities we have and sanctifies them for his purposes, or he bestows on us spiritual gifts that lead us out of a general healing ministry into a particular branch of it.

So, for example, one of the team may decide they want to become more skilled in counselling. They begin by joining a Christian Listeners course, such as that run by the Acorn Christian Healing Trust, and then go on to qualify as counsellors with the Association of Christian Counsellors or some such institution. Dioceses and other district and provincial bodies are always on the lookout for suitable counsellors to whom they can refer troubled clergy and church leaders.

In one parish a married couple formed a charitable trust and, with a group of part-time assistants and the support of their congregation, set up a counselling service that was soon serving increasing numbers every day of the week.

The church's healing prayer team found this a valuable resource for they were able to commend to the trust individuals whose problems were too deep-seated for the team to handle.

In another parish a small group also formed a charitable trust to purchase a large house and, with some members living in it as a community and others committing themselves to join them on certain days each week, offered residential care for those who need personal support for short periods. There are numbers of similar initiatives, many of them ecumenical, all over the country.

There is a saying that Christians do not always see eye to eye together, but they can walk arm in arm. Those involved in communities and other closely knit groups almost inevitably run into trouble through personality clashes or internal disputes about policy. These upsets cannot always be avoided, but steps can be taken to help them overcome such difficulties if and when they arise.

First, when a group or community is set up for a specialist ministry, it has to be clear what its aims are (these are roughly the equivalent of the rules that govern the life of a traditional religious order). These aims are finalized after prayer and reflection on God's purposes for them, and after frank discussion among potential members. The aims are written down and form the basis of a community covenant to which all members commit themselves. This covenant then becomes a reference point when questions and disagreements about policies arise. In time it may be right to modify or change this covenant, but that is only done with the consent of the community (and of the board of trustees, if there is one).

Second, it is a condition of membership that they pray together regularly. In the case of a residential community this should be at least daily. Unless the ministry of these groups and communities is undergirded with prayer, members will soon find themselves at odds with one another, and at worst their work will cease to be distinctly Christian. Within the rule of prayer there is an agreement about receiving Communion together, either in church or in the house.

Third, a board of Christians who are sympathetic to the aims of the group or of the community is formed. They are invaluable as advisers and intercessors, doubling up as trustees if charitable status is called for. When the kinds of difficulties just mentioned occur, it is to this board that the group or community appeals for advice.

The Charity Commissioners require trusts to submit a copy of charities' audited accounts to be sent to them at intervals, so it is useful if one of the trustees can act as treasurer or financial adviser. The sort of individual required for this job is one who has accountancy skills but who also understands why Christians with little in the bank sometimes have to launch out on a project trusting in the Lord's provision!

Fourth and finally, a wider network of supporters beyond the advisers and trustees – often given the title of Friends – helps groups and communities to develop their ministry. The Friends receive newsletters and prayer requests. They are invited to special events. They may also be willing to respond to appeals for practical help or financial assistance from time to time. In the case of residential communities, Friends can also help the community not become too inward-looking.

The statutory social services and other caring professions can be helpful to these groups and communities, though they do not always appreciate the vision that has brought these Christians together. When I was a member of the Barnabas Fellowship at Whatcombe House in Dorset (which grew out of a church prayer group in Essex) we had to learn to be wise as serpents and harmless as doves about our relationships with them.

The Fellowship consisted of a dozen or so who believed that the Lord had called us to live in the large Georgian manor as a praying community with a ministry to help Christians and their churches to seek renewal in the Holy Spirit. It was a vision we pursued through week-long, weekend, and midweek residential conferences. It was a demanding and exhausting ministry – we had up to 2,000 guests a year – and we found we had to guard strictly those periods when we were closed to visitors in order to recover our strength and do practical jobs round the house.

The local social services soon heard about us and decided that, as a group of Christians, we were bound to welcome some of their more difficult cases, particularly folk whom, they thought, would benefit from living in the countryside with a family-like group for several weeks. Initially we accepted two or three of their cases. These were individuals with great needs, and we did what we could for them; but we soon realized that they occupied so much of our time and energy (and prayers!) that we were being diverted from the work to which we believed God had called us.

After much soul-searching (did the Lord want us to change our aims?) we resolved that we must refuse to accept further cases. No doubt the social services thought we were very unchristian, but time showed that we had made the right decision. Groups and communities must be faithful to their original vision and refuse to be diverted from it, unless their experiences lead them to believe that the vision has to be changed.

I have known a few Christian men and women who, after being members of a healing prayer team, have left their jobs to train as doctors, nurses and other care workers as a result of what they have experienced through the team's ministry.

Some of the developments I have described may only last for a few years. Whatcombe itself had to close after 14 years (though that was because the house would no longer be approved by the county fire service as a conference centre, not because there was a lack of demand for its ministry). But such terminations are not necessarily a sign of failure. Groups and communities, like human beings, seem to have a certain lifespan and then fade away. They fulfil the Lord's work during the years of their existence, and then their members scatter to be used by him elsewhere. What they have experienced is not lost; it has enriched their personal growth in Christ and prepared them for their future ministries.

For Discussion

- Have you ever visited a community in which the ministry of healing is exercised? If so, what did you think and feel about it afterwards?
- Do you envisage yourself being involved in a ministry of healing that is wider than that offered in your local church?

POSTSCRIPT

Some years ago a local Churches Together committee invited
me to preach at a united service during the Week of Prayer
for Christian Unity. They asked me to preach on the subject
of Christian healing. When I arrived I was pleasantly surprised to find the building filled with between 150 and 200
people. After a time of worship, led by a group of musicians
(drawn together for the occasion from different churches),
scripture readings and prayers, I went in the pulpit.

I gave a general introduction to the subject and described
how different churches were exercising the healing ministry.
Towards the end I felt as if the Holy Spirit was nudging me
to follow up what I was saying by offering to pray with any
who had been stirred by what I said. Initially I was appalled
at the idea. What would happen if many responded? Then I
comforted myself with the thought that perhaps only one or
two would come forward, so at the end of the sermon I gave
the invitation. To my dismay it seemed as if about a quarter
of those present were raising their hands.

In a flash it seemed as if I received a further instruction:
'Ask for helpers.' So I did. 'Are there any here who regularly
pray with others for healing in their churches?' I enquired.
To my immense relief about a dozen other hands went up.

Descending from the pulpit, I beckoned this dozen forward, gave them brief instructions and divided them into
pairs. They began ministering to individuals at stations
in different parts of the church while the music group

gently sang choruses. I returned to the pulpit to oversee the proceedings.

It was then that I realized I was witnessing a minor near-miracle. Here was an Anglican paired with a Methodist, there was a Roman Catholic paired with a Baptist, and over there was a United Reformed Church member paired with a New Church member. Other ecumenical pairings were spread round the church. They were welcoming individuals, listening to them, laying hands on them and praying with them, as if they had been doing it together for ages.

The lesson went home to my heart as well as my mind: when Christians from different traditions yield to the unity they have in Jesus Christ, the gifts of the Holy Spirit that he distributes among them bring even greater glory to God. That ecumenical congregation had truly become 'a touching place'.

Book List

Percy Dearmer, *The Parson's Handbook* (1907), Oxford University Press, 1965.

John Gunstone, *Healed, Restored, Forgiven: Liturgies, Prayers and Readings for the Ministry of Healing*, Canterbury Press, 2004.

George Hacker, *The Healing Stream: Catholic Insights into the Ministry of Healing*, Darton, Longman and Todd, 1998.

John Leach, *Person Centred Prayer Ministry*, Grove Books, 2002.

Francis MacNutt, *Healing*, Hodder & Stoughton, 1997.

Russ Parker, Derek Fraser and David Rivers, *In Search of Wholeness: A Christian Theology of Healing and Practical Training for Church and Medical Settings*, St John's Extension Studies, Bramcote, Nottingham NG9 3RL, 2003.

J. Cameron Peddie, *The Forgotten Talent* (1942), Arthur James, 1985.

Tom Smail, *Windows on the Cross*, Darton, Longman and Todd, 1995.

A Time to Heal: A Report to the House of Bishops on the Healing Ministry, Church House Publishing, 2000.

Roger Vaughan, *Saints Alive! Healing in the Church* (revised edition of *Saints for Healing*), Resource, 4 Old Station Yard, Abingdon, Oxfordshire OX14 3LD, 2004.

Keith Warrington, *Jesus the Healer: Paradigm or Unique Phenomenon?*, Paternoster Press, 2000.

John Wimber and Kevin Springer, *Power Healing*, Hodder & Stoughton, 1986/2001.

Websites

www.burrswood.org.uk

www.cofe.anglican.org/worship/liturgy/commonworship
For the texts of the ministry of healing and wholeness.

www.ccr.org.uk
Catholic Charismatic Renewal's website with links to Roman Catholic resources, including 'Healing'.

www.methodist-central-hall.org.uk/healing

www.guild-of-st-raphael.org.uk

www.acornchristian.org.uk

www.gohealth.org.uk
Guild of Health.

www.leeabbey.org.uk

www.cmf.org.uk
Christian Medical Fellowship.

A search on the web for 'The Church's Ministry of Healing' (or something similar) produces about 200,000 sites. However, some national and provincial ecclesiastical offices have useful links. One of these links is in the website of the Chichester diocese:

www.diochi.org.uk/content/support/mission/healing.htm

INDEX OF SUBJECTS